Pegan Diet

"Eat Better, Feel Better: 100 Guide to Eating Pegan for Optimal Health and Wellness"

Richy Moss

Copyright (c) [2022] by [RICHY MOSS]

The information contained in this book is for general information purposes only. The author has made every effort to ensure the accuracy of the information contained in this book, but does not assume any liability for errors or omissions. The author and publisher specifically disclaim any and all liability for any claims or damages that may result from the use of the information contained in this book.

This book is not intended as a substitute for professional advice. If you require legal, financial, or other professional advice, you should seek the services of a qualified professional.

The author and publisher of this book do not assume any responsibility for any errors or omissions, nor do they assume any liability for any injuries or damages arising from the use of the information contained in this book.

TABLE OF CONTENT

INTRODUCTION TO A PEGAN DIET COOK BOOK 4

CHAPTER ONE 7

    BREAKFAST COOKBOOK RECIPES FOR A PEGAN DIET. 7

        THE BENEFIT OF BACON AND EGG MUFFIN TO HEALTH 13

CHAPTER TWO 25

    RECIPES FOR A PEGAN DEIT LUNCH. 25

    WHAT ARE THE HEALTH BENEFITS OF A PEGAN DIET BOOK'S LUNCH RECIPES. 26

CHAPTER THREE 37

    AN OVERVIEW OF THE DINNER DIET 37

    PRINCIPLE #1: ROASTED VEGGIES AND CHICKEN FOR A PALEO DIET. 38

CHAPTER 4 64

    INTRODUCTION 64

        PRINCIPLE #2 66

    OVERVIEW 70

    BENEFITS OF ROASTED NUTS FOR A PALEO DIET 70

CHAPTER 5 79

    INTRODUCTION TO DESSERT RECIPES FOR A PEGAN DIET. 79

    PRINCIPLE #1: APPLE CRISP PEGAN DIET 81

    PRINCIPLE 2: PALEO BROWNIES 82

    PRINCIPLE #3 89

    INTRODUCTION 89

INTRODUCTION TO A PEGAN DIET COOK BOOK

Greetings and welcome to the Paleo-Vegan Cookbook! This in-depth manual was created to assist you in following the guidelines of the Paleo-Vegan diet while preparing meals that are scrumptious and nourishing. The Paleo-Vegan diet is an original fusion of two of the most well-liked health and wellness fads in existence right now: the Paleo diet and the Vegan diet. Consuming whole, unprocessed foods that are as close to their natural state as possible is encouraged by the Paleo diet. The vegan diet emphasizes plant-based foods and forbids the consumption of any animal products. Combining these two diets gives you a diet that is high in beneficial proteins and fats and low in processed foods, giving you the best of both worlds..

The Paleo-Vegan Diet Cookbook is brimming with delectable recipes that are easy to make. The pages that follow provide a range of recipes for breakfast, lunch, dinner, snacks, and dessert. Every recipe is made to provide you with the maximum amount of nourishment while maintaining the flavors of your favorite foods. You'll have everything you need to start preparing delectable vegan and paleo-friendly meals with the aid of this book. Let's get cooking right away!

Combining the Paleo and vegan diets, the Pegan diet is a style of eating that is becoming more and more well-liked. It places an emphasis on a plant-based diet that includes lots of fruits, vegetables, nuts, and seeds while also allowing for small amounts of animal protein such that found in fish, chicken, and eggs. This diet is intended to encourage weight loss, enhance general health, and lessen inflammatory responses inside the body.

The Pegan diet is based on the idea that processed and refined foods should generally be avoided because they are frequently rich in sugar and fat and lacking in nutrients. A concentration on complete, unprocessed foods that are high in vitamins, minerals, and healthy fats is encouraged by the diet. Fruits, vegetables, whole grains, nuts, and seeds are some of these foods.

The Pegan diet is based on the premise that most processed and refined foods should be avoided, as they are often low in nutrients and high in unhealthy fats and sugar. Instead, the diet encourages people to focus on whole, unprocessed foods that are rich in vitamins, minerals, and healthy fats. These foods include fruits, vegetables, whole grains, nuts, seeds, legumes, and healthy oils.

In addition to these whole foods, the Pegan diet also allows for moderate amounts of lean proteins, such as poultry, eggs, and fish. However, red meat, dairy, and processed meats are to be avoided. Sugary beverages, such as soda and energy drinks, as well as refined grains, are also off-limits.

The Pegan diet also permits modest amounts of lean proteins like chicken, eggs, and fish in addition to these complete foods. Red meat, dairy products, and processed meats should be avoided. Refined carbohydrates and sugary drinks like soda and energy drinks are also forbidden.

The Pegan diet focuses on nutrient-dense, whole foods that are naturally low in calories and is a fantastic method to lose weight and enhance health. This type of eating also lowers inflammation, which can help lower the chance of developing chronic illnesses like diabetes and heart disease.

The Pegan diet is a fantastic way to eat for both health and weight loss overall. By emphasizing complete, unadulterated meals and keeping portion sizes small.

CHAPTER ONE
BREAKFAST COOKBOOK RECIPES FOR A PEGAN DIET.

The most significant meal of the day is breakfast, so it's crucial to have a filling and delectable meal to start the day. There are many breakfast options available, whether you're following the Paleo diet or a variation of it, like the Pegan diet. There is something for everyone, from savory egg dishes to recipes that are suitable for vegans.

When it comes to breakfast, eggs are always a fantastic option. Breakfast burritos, frittatas, and omelets may all be quickly prepared to be tasty and nutritious. If you eat a vegan diet, you can substitute a tofu scramble with vegetables for the eggs.

Breakfast casseroles are an additional well-liked choice. Whether it's a traditional egg bake or a sweet potato and kale casserole, these recipes are easy to prepare and can be prepared ahead of time for a quick meal.

Make your own Paleo-friendly granola if you're searching for something a little sweeter. This is a fantastic way to obtain your daily serving of protein and good fats in the morning. A smoothie bowl can also be created with a variety of fruits, nuts, and seeds.

Last but not least, don't overlook breakfast sandwiches. Vegan ingredients such as tempeh bacon and vegan cheese can be used to make a traditional egg sandwich. Make a French toast-style sandwich with nut butter and fruit for a sweeter lunch.

Whatever type of breakfast you prefer, there are many delectable and wholesome options for the Pegan diet. You can make a filling and delectable breakfast that will get your day started right with a little imagination and a few basic items.

For the Pegan diet, here are some more breakfast suggestions:

• Coconut yogurt parfait with nuts, seeds, and fresh fruit • Overnight oats with nut butter and banana slices • Sweet potato toast with avocado and smoked salmon

Egg muffins with veggies and herbs; Veggie omelets with vegan cheese; Spinach and mushroom frittata; Banana and nut butter breakfast cookies; Sweet potato hash with crispy bacon and eggs; Chia pudding; Paleo-friendly pancakes with almond butter and fresh berries.

Examples:

1. Bacon and egg muffins: A delicious way to start the day is with bacon and egg muffins. They are quick and simple to prepare and may be done in advance for an easy breakfast. Pre-heat your oven to 375 degrees before making them. Each muffin cup should have a bacon slice in it after greasing the pan.

2. Sweet Potato Hash: A protein-rich breakfast that will keep you full until lunchtime is sweet potato hash. It is prepared by heating some oil in a skillet over medium-high heat. Sweet potatoes cubed should be added and cooked until they start to soften. Add the onion, garlic, and bell peppers in dice and sauté until the vegetables are soft. Add the diced cooked bacon last, followed by the salt and pepper.

3. Paleo pancakes: Pancakes are a classic morning food that don't always have to be harmful. Almond flour, tapioca flour, and baking powder should be combined in a bowl to make a Paleo variation. Combine eggs, almond milk, coconut oil, and honey in another bowl. Stirring is required after adding the wet ingredients to the dry ones. Some oil in a skillet is heated to medium-high heat. The batter should be poured into the skillet and cooked until golden. Serve with your preferred garnishes.

4. Tuna Salad: Tuna salad makes a delightful breakfast in addition to being a fantastic lunch or dinner choice. To create it, combine canned tuna, sliced onion, celery, and mustard in a bowl along with the mayo, mustard, and lemon juice. Serve with your preferred crackers or on top of a bed of mixed greens, then season with salt and pepper.

5. Greek salad: If you're looking for a healthy and light breakfast, a Greek salad can be a terrific choice. Cucumber, tomato, red onion, and olives sliced are combined in a bowl to produce it. Olive oil and feta cheese are used as garnish. Toast made from whole wheat is served alongside.

6. Turkey Sliders: Turkey sliders are a fantastic breakfast option for getting your protein. Pre-heat your oven to 375 degrees before making them. In a bowl, mix the seasonings, minced onion, minced garlic, and ground turkey. Make tiny patties out of the mixture, then bake them for 20 minutes, or until fully done. Serve with your preferred dipping sauce on slider buns.

7. Chicken with Roasted Veggies: A quick and wholesome breakfast option as well as a dinner option. Set your oven's temperature to 425. Organize the vegetables and diced chicken on a baking sheet. Add olive oil on top.

8. Salmon with coconut rice: As a rich source of protein and good fats, salmon is a fantastic choice for breakfast. Cook the salmon for 4-5 minutes on each side in a skillet that has been heated to medium-high heat. Cook some coconut rice in a different pan in accordance with the directions on the package. Serve the fish with your favorite vegetables and the coconut rice.

When the mozzarella cheese is melted and bubbling, bake for another 25 minutes. With a side of salad, please.

10. Paleo trail mix: In addition to being a terrific snack, trail mix also makes a tasty breakfast. It is made by mixing dark chocolate chips, almonds, walnuts, pumpkin seeds, and sunflower seeds in a bowl. For a quick and simple breakfast, combine all the ingredients and store in an airtight container. With a glass of almond milk, serve.

11. Zucchini Fries: Having zucchini fries for breakfast is a terrific way to obtain your daily serving of vegetables. Set your oven at 425 degrees and get to work making them. Slice a zucchini into fries-like pieces, then arrange the fries on a baking pan. Saturate with salt and pepper and drizzle with olive oil. 20 to 25 minutes of baking, or until golden brown. Serve with a side of ketchup or ranch dressing

12. Roasted Nuts: A fantastic approach to acquire good fats in the morning is by eating roasted nuts. Set your oven at 350 degrees and get to work making them. On a baking sheet, scatter your preferred nuts

(almonds, walnuts, cashews, etc.) and season with salt, pepper, and a little olive oil. 8 to 10 minutes of baking, or until golden brown. Snack on it or sprinkle it over your breakfast.

13. Apple Crisp: Apple crisp is a tasty and nutritious dessert that is a simple morning option. Set your oven to 375 degrees and get to work making it. Apples should be cored, sliced, and put in a baking dish. Add a layer of melted butter, almond flour, and oats on top. Bake for 25 minutes, or until golden brown on top.

14. Paleo Brownies: Brownies may not be the first thing you think of for breakfast, but these Paleo-friendly brownies are a great way to enjoy a sweet treat in the morning. To make them, preheat your oven to 350 degrees. Mix together almond butter, eggs, coconut sugar, cocoa powder, and baking powder in a bowl. Pour the batter into a greased baking dish and bake for 20-25 minutes or until a toothpick inserted into the center comes out clean.

15. Coconut Macaroons: A tasty and simple dessert that is great for breakfast are coconut macaroons. To make them, combine egg whites, almond flour, coconut sugar, and finely chopped coconut in a bowl. Create little balls out of the mixture, then set them on a baking sheet. Until golden brown, bake for 12 to 15 minutes. Enjoy as a snack or a topping for Greek yogurt or porridge.

EGG AND BACON MUFFINS

For those following a Paleo diet, bacon and egg muffins are a quick, simple, and delectable breakfast choice. In this recipe, bacon and eggs, two traditional breakfast components, are combined to create a delicious and wholesome muffin. The outcome is a flavorful, protein-rich breakfast that is portable.

High-quality bacon, preferably pasture-raised and devoid of nitrates and preservatives, serves as the foundation of this recipe. After being cooked until crispy, the bacon is crumbled and added to the muffin pan. After being immediately broken into the tin, the eggs are cooked until set. The end result is a flavorful and delicious muffin that is high in protein.

By altering the egg muffins, any dietary restriction or palate preference can be satisfied. To add sweetness, think about adding some diced apples or pears. For more crunch, stir in additional chopped nuts or seeds. Adding some diced avocado or crumbled sausage could also help to increase the amount of protein and good fats in the dish.

Warm egg muffins go best with fresh fruit or a salad on the side. They are excellent for breakfast on-the-go or as a component of a bigger breakfast presentation. The muffins can be prepared ahead of time and kept for up to three days in the refrigerator. Simply microwave them for a little period of time, or bake them in the oven until warm.

These bacon and egg muffins will satisfy your need for either a speedy breakfast or a handy snack.

Enjoy!

THE BENEFIT OF BACON AND EGG MUFFIN TO HEALTH

This muffin recipe's inclusion of bacon and eggs has several health advantages. Protein, good fats, and vital vitamins and minerals can all be found in plenty in bacon. Additionally, eggs are a good source of protein and are rich in key vitamins, minerals, and choline, which is crucial for maintaining brain health. A nutrient-dense breakfast or snack that combines these two components into a single muffin will help you stay nourished and energized all day.

BENEFITS OF THE MENU

- Quick and simple to prepare

- Excellent grab-and-go breakfast

- Get it in advance and kept in the refrigerator

- Versatile and adaptable to varied components

- Rich in healthy fats and protein

- Packed with necessary vitamins and minerals

- Can be a part of a bigger breakfast spread - Lightweight and portable - Delicious and satisfying - Ideal for active lives.

DISADVANTAGES

There are a few possible drawbacks to bacon and egg muffins, despite the fact that they can be a quick and wholesome supper. Bacon should only be eaten seldom because it contains a lot of saturated fat and salt. Salmonella contamination is also a possibility because the eggs are baked in a muffin pan. Use pasteurized eggs whenever feasible to reduce this danger.

SUGAR COATED POTATOES FOR A PEGAN DIET

A delicious and healthy breakfast option, sweet potato hash is a terrific way to start the day. Due to its abundance of nutritious ingredients, it is ideal for people who follow the Paleo or Pegan diets. A flavor combination that is difficult to top is produced by the blending of sweet potatoes, onions, peppers, and spices.

This meal may be tailored to any taste and is really simple to prepare. Furthermore, it's a fantastic way to use up any leftover vegetables you might have in the fridge. While the onions and peppers offer a healthy serving of fiber and vitamins, the sweet potatoes are a fantastic source of complex carbohydrates.

To prepare this recipe, you must first preheat your oven to 375 degrees. Chop the sweet potatoes into cubes after peeling them. On a baking sheet, arrange the cubes and sprinkle them with a mixture of your preferred herbs and spices. After that, combine a little olive oil, salt, and pepper with the potatoes. For around 20 minutes, roast the potatoes in the oven.

Heat a sizable skillet over medium heat once the potatoes have been roasted. Add the onions and peppers after adding a tablespoon of olive oil. Till they are soft, sauce the vegetables for around 5 minutes. Cook the roasted sweet potatoes in the pan for a further five minutes. Add any more seasonings you like to finish.

The best way to start your day is with this sweet potato hash. It has a ton of taste and is a fantastic source of complex carbs and fiber. It is a versatile dish because the vegetables can be changed to your preferences. You will undoubtedly adore it whether you consume it hot or cold.

How To Prepare This Menu Examples;

A delicious and simple breakfast option for individuals on a Paleo or Pegan diet is sweet potato hash. Here is a detailed recipe for this delectable dish.

In the first step, heat the oven to 375 degrees.

Step 2: Cut the sweet potatoes into cubes after peeling them. On a baking sheet, arrange the cubes and sprinkle them with a mixture of your preferred herbs and spices.

Step 3: Add some olive oil, a bit of salt, and some pepper to the potatoes.

Step 4: Roast the potatoes for 20 minutes or so in the oven.

5. Turn a big skillet to medium heat. Add the onions and peppers after adding a tablespoon of olive oil. Till they are soft, sauce the vegetables for around 5 minutes.

The roasted sweet potatoes should be added to the pan in step 6 and cooked for an additional 5 minutes.

Step 7: Add any other seasonings you want to the dish.

Step 8: Whether hot or cold, serve the sweet potato hash. Enjoy!

MENU'S HEALTH BENEFIT

In addition to being a fantastic source of fiber and complex carbohydrates, sweet potato hash is also a good source of vitamins and minerals. Sweet potatoes have B vitamins, potassium, and magnesium and are a strong source of vitamins A and C. Additionally good sources of vitamins, minerals, and dietary fiber include peppers and onions. This dish is a fantastic source of antioxidants, which can aid in illness prevention. The used olive oil also has beneficial fats and can aid in lowering inflammation in the body.

For those who follow a Paleo or Pegan diet, sweet potato hash is a wonderful and filling dish. It is a fantastic way to start the day and may be tailored to your preferences. Furthermore, it's a fantastic way to use up any leftover vegetables you might have in the fridge. A flavor combination that is difficult to top is produced by the blending of sweet potatoes, onions, peppers, and spices. In addition, this recipe is exceedingly simple to create and takes only a few minutes. You will definitely enjoy this dish whether you eat it hot or cold, so make sure to do so.

PEGAN DIET BOOK: PALEO PANCAKES

A delightful and wholesome way to start your day is with Paleo pancakes. These pancakes, which are made with almond flour, coconut milk, and eggs, are not only flavorful and satisfying to eat but also a good source of protein and healthy fats. These gluten-free, dairy-free, and nutrient-rich pancakes are ideal for people following the Paleo diet.

Start by mixing the baking powder, salt, cinnamon, and almond flour in a sizable basin. Combine the eggs, coconut milk, melted butter, and honey in another bowl. Stir after each addition of the wet ingredients until just mixed.

Spray cooking spray onto a non-stick skillet and heat it up over medium heat. Pour 1/4 cup of batter into the skillet and heat until the center is bubbly and the sides are golden brown. Cook for two more minutes after flipping. Use the leftover batter to repeat.

Fresh fruit, nut butter, or even a sprinkle of honey can be added to Paleo pancakes as toppings. They go well with a variety of side dishes, including sautéed veggies, bacon, and eggs. Enjoy your Paleo pancakes with a filling breakfast to get your day started off right.

WHO CAN MAKE PALEO?

A growing number of people are adopting the paleolithic diet, which emphasizes consuming entire, unprocessed foods that are as close to their original forms as possible. It is based on the Paleolithic diet of our ancestors, which included various meats, fish, nuts, seeds, fruits, and vegetables.

The Paleo diet is rich in nutrients and provides them from foods like eggs, nuts, seeds, and fruits as well as other necessary vitamins and minerals. It is also highly well-balanced, with a focus on protein, low-glycemic carbohydrates, and healthy fats. It promotes eating largely organic, grass-fed, and wild-caught foods and is free of gluten, dairy, and other processed foods.

The fact that the Paleo diet is very anti-inflammatory is one of its key advantages. Eliminating refined carbohydrates and processed meals reduces inflammation in the body, which benefits a number of chronic health disorders. Additionally, it aids in weight loss since it lessens cravings and prolongs feelings of fullness.

The Paleo diet is a fantastic way to eat a balanced diet that is rich in wholesome foods with amazing flavors. It is a great option for people who want to get healthier overall, decrease weight, and reduce inflammation.

In conclusion, anyone seeking a nutritious and well-balanced diet should strongly consider the Paleo diet. Because it is free of processed foods and refined sugars, inflammation is reduced, and overall health may be improved. It promotes consuming organic, grass-fed, and wild-caught foods while offering vital vitamins and minerals. You can enjoy scrumptious and healthy meals while enhancing your general health by adhering to the Paleo diet.

HOW CAN THE PALEO DIET BENEFIT THE CIRCULATORY AND DIGESTIVE SYSTEMS?

The Paleo diet promotes the eating of nutrient-dense foods that are simple to digest, which benefits the circulatory and digestive systems. The diet excludes dairy, grains, legumes, and processed foods, which are frequently hard to digest and can inflame the digestive tract. The Paleo diet also contains a lot of fiber, which benefits in the absorption of nutrients and the promotion of regular bowel movements.

The Paleo diet also supports the maintenance of a healthy circulatory system by supplying vital nutrients including Vitamin B12, Folate, Iron, and Magnesium. These nutrients and vitamins promote circulation and guard against anemia, which keeps the circulatory system functioning properly. The diet also contains a lot of omega-3 fatty acids, which are known to reduce inflammation and improve blood pressure and heart health.

DISCUSS THE ACTIONS REQUIRED TO SET UP A PALEO DIET

1. Eliminate Processed Foods: Eliminating processed foods is the first step in planning a Paleo diet. Foods like white flour, refined sugar, artificial sweeteners, and processed vegetable oils fall under this category.

2. Consume Whole Foods: The next stage is to concentrate on consuming as many whole, unadulterated foods as you can. This includes fresh fruits and vegetables, grass-fed cattle, free-range chicken, wild-caught fish, and healthy fats like avocados, olive oil, and coconut oil.

3. Include Healthy Fats: Healthy fats are a crucial component of a Paleo diet since they offer critical vitamins and minerals and can fight inflammation. These fats come in various forms, such as olive oil, coconut oil, avocados, nuts, and seeds.

4. Consume Lots of Vegetables: Considering how low in calories and high in vitamins and minerals vegetables are, they should make up a significant portion of a Paleo diet. Aim to consume 5 servings or more of vegetables each day.

5. Include Healthy Proteins: Healthy proteins are a crucial component of the Paleo diet and include grass-fed beef, free-range chicken, wild-caught fish, and eggs. They give you critical vitamins and minerals and support your ability to feel content and full.

6. Avoid Refined Sugars: When following the Paleo diet, refined sugars should be avoided because they might promote inflammation and weight gain. Choose natural sweeteners like honey, maple syrup, and coconut sugar instead.

7. Maintain Hydration: Maintaining proper hydration is crucial for maintaining good body function when on the Paleo diet. Try to drink 8 glasses of water or more each day.

8. Get Enough Sleep: Sleep is crucial to your overall health and happiness. Try to obtain 7-8 hours of good sleep every night.

HOW CAN A PALEO DIET ASSIST YOU IN WEIGHT LOSS

Because it excludes processed foods, refined carbohydrates, and harmful fats, a Paleo diet can aid in weight loss. This aids in calorie restriction, desire reduction, and weight loss. The diet is also rich in protein and good fats, which can help you feel satisfied and full for extended periods of time. Consuming a range of nutrient-dense foods can help to deliver important vitamins and minerals and maintain a healthy metabolism. The emphasis on whole, unprocessed foods also encourage this. Last but not least, a diet high in fiber encourages regular bowel motions and helps the body absorb nutrients. Combining each of these elements can support weight loss and a healthier way of life.

A Paleo diet can aid in weight loss as well as bettering general health and wellbeing. The foods that are high in nutrients can aid in supplying important vitamins and minerals and reducing inflammation. In addition, cutting out processed meals and refined sugars can lower your risk of developing chronic illnesses like diabetes and heart disease. Finally, putting an emphasis on complete, unprocessed foods may aid with digestion, bloating, and other digestive problems. Together, all of these elements may support greater general health.

ADVANTAGES OF A PALEO DIET FOR HEALTH

THE PALEO DIET HAS MANY HEALTH BENEFITS, LIKE:

1. Reducing inflammation: Processed foods, refined carbohydrates, and bad fats are all prohibited on the Paleo diet because they can increase inflammation in the body. As a result of reducing inflammation, chronic diseases including diabetes, heart disease, and cancer can be avoided.

2. Rich in important vitamins and minerals: The Paleo diet is full of nutritious, wholesome foods that supply important vitamins and minerals. The body needs certain vitamins and minerals to function at its best and to potentially boost general health.

3. Improving digestion: The Paleo diet is strong in fiber, which aids in the absorption of nutrients and helps to encourage regular bowel movements. Additionally, bloating and other digestive problems can be lessened by cutting out processed foods and refined sugars.

4. Weight Loss: Due to its ability to suppress cravings and keep you feeling full and satisfied for longer periods of time, the Paleo diet can help you lose weight.

5. Enhanced energy levels: The Paleo diet is rich in healthy fats and proteins that can help you feel more energised all day long.

In summary, the Paleo diet has several health benefits, including lowering inflammation, supplying vital vitamins and minerals, enhancing digestion, encouraging weight loss, and boosting energy. It is a great option for anyone who want to enhance their general health and wellbeing.

HOW CAN A VEGETARIAN BENEFIT FROM A PEGAN DIET?

By offering a balanced diet that includes both plant-based and animal-based foods, the Pegan diet can benefit a vegetarian. The Pegan diet, which emphasizes eating largely plant-based meals with some animal-based foods as well, is a cross between the Paleo and Vegan diets. Variety of fruits and vegetables, nuts and seeds, good fats, and trace amounts of animal-based proteins like fish and eggs are all included in it.

For vegetarians who want to supplement their diet with things other than plants, the Pegan diet is a fantastic option. Along with beneficial proteins, lipids, and carbohydrates, it also supplies vital vitamins and minerals. It is also free of refined carbohydrates, bad fats, and processed foods, all of which can assist to lower inflammation and support a healthy lifestyle.

The Pegan diet offers vegetarians a balanced diet that contains both plant-based and animal-based items, which, in turn, can be helpful for them. Along with beneficial proteins, lipids, and carbohydrates, it also supplies vital vitamins and minerals. It is also free of refined carbohydrates, bad fats, and processed foods, all of which can assist to lower inflammation and support a healthy lifestyle.

CHAPTER TWO

RECIPES FOR A PEGAN DEIT LUNCH.

Any healthy diet must include lunch, and the Paleo diet is no exception. Consuming a healthy lunch gives you the energy you need to stay alert and productive throughout the rest of the day. Here are some mouthwatering options that are sure to please if you're looking for some tasty and healthy lunch recipes to add to your Paleo diet plan.

A traditional lunch option that is flavorful and simple to prepare is tuna salad. To begin, put diced celery, diced red onion, diced bell pepper, and canned tuna in a bowl. Add a tablespoon of lemon juice and extra virgin olive oil, and then season with salt and pepper to taste. Serve in a wrap for a take-along lunch or on top of a bed of fresh greens.

Greek Salad is an additional delectable lunch option. Cucumber, red onion, cherry tomatoes, and pitted Kalamata olives should first be combined in a bowl. Add oregano, salt, and pepper to taste, then drizzle with a tablespoon of extra virgin olive oil and a tablespoon of red wine vinegar. For a flavorful and healthy lunch, serve with feta cheese crumbled on the side.

A simple and delicious lunch option that can be made quickly is turkey sliders. In a bowl, first combine ground turkey with diced onion, bell pepper, and one clove of minced garlic. Small patties made from the mixture should be cooked in a lightly greased skillet at medium heat. Serve on a toasted whole wheat bread with a piece of tomato and a slice of lettuce on top of each burger.

These are only a handful of the mouthwatering lunch recipes you may include in your Paleo diet regimen. These dishes are all packed with healthy ingredients and are certain to sate any appetite. These Paleo-friendly meals are sure to please, whether you're searching for a quick lunch to get you through the afternoon or a big dinner to keep you motivated all day.

WHAT ARE THE HEALTH BENEFITS OF A PEGAN DIET BOOK'S LUNCH RECIPES.

Lunch meals for a Pegan Diet Book include a variety of health advantages. These dishes often contain a lot of protein and fiber, which helps you feel full and satisfied for a longer period of time. In addition to reducing cravings and keeping you energized all day, eating a healthy lunch can assist to balance your blood sugar levels. Getting the vitamins and minerals your body requires to stay strong and healthy can also be accomplished by eating a balanced lunch. These recipes are also frequently low in bad fats and added sugar, making them a wonderful option for anyone trying to keep their weight in check.

These lunch ideas are also delicious and simple to make, which makes them a fantastic option for people who are busy and don't have a lot of time to spend in the kitchen. Last but not least, lunch recipes from a Pegan Diet Book are frequently free of gluten, dairy, and processed ingredients, making them a fantastic option for anyone who have food sensitivities or are on a particular diet.

SALAD TUNA FOR PEGAN.

A tasty, healthful lunch may be had with tuna salad without feeling like you're compromising flavor. This recipe is suitable for paleo and vegan diets and is loaded with vegetables, healthy fats, and protein for a filling lunch or light dinner. It is simple to make and may be tailored to your preferences.

Start by mixing cooked tuna, diced cooked potatoes, and diced celery in a bowl to prepare the salad. Add some chopped scallions, dill, and parsley after that. You can add some paleo mayonnaise for a creamy texture. You can add capers and lemon juice for flavor if you'd like. Add salt and pepper to the salad as a final touch.

You may get all the health advantages of tuna without having to eat it plain by adding it to a salad. It is the perfect paleo and vegan supper because it is heavy in protein and low in fat. Omega-3 fatty acids, which have been demonstrated to lessen inflammation in the body and may aid in lowering cholesterol levels, are also abundant in it. Additionally, selenium, which is essential for thyroid health and can help prevent cancer, is a wonderful source of nutrition in tuna.

This salad is a fantastic method to increase the amount of vegetables in your diet. The celery, parsley, and scallions give fantastic flavor, and the diced potatoes and potatoes offer some nice crunch. Additionally, you may always add some additional vegetables of your choosing.

A quick and simple lunch that works for any day of the week is tuna salad. It's ideal for meal preparation, allowing you to quickly prepare a nutritious lunch or dinner. For a full dinner, serve it alone or with a side of greens.

WHAT TO DO TO PREPARE IT AND WHAT STEPS NEED TO BE TAKEN.

Cooked tuna, diced cooked potatoes, diced celery, chopped parsley, dill, scallions, paleo mayonnaise, lemon juice, capers, salt, and pepper are all ingredients needed to make tuna salad. In a bowl, first combine each ingredient. After that, combine everything and stir until the ingredients are dispersed equally. Add salt and pepper to taste and finish by seasoning the salad.

It's crucial to use canned tuna that has been packed in water rather than oil when making tuna salad. This will assist in reducing the salad's fat content. In order to prevent the salad from becoming overly watery, take sure to drain the tuna before adding it. To ensure that the dish adheres to the vegan and paleo diets, use mayonnaise that is suitable for these diets.

SERVING RECOMMENDATIONS AND MODIFICATIONS

You can serve tuna salad either by itself or with a side of greens. You may serve it on a bed of lettuce or in a wrap because it also works well as a sandwich filling. Add some cooked quinoa or brown rice for a heartier supper. Avocado slices can be added to the salad as a topping for more taste and nutrition.

You can make tuna salad to your preferences. You are welcome to include more vegetables of your choice. Additionally, you can change the seasonings to your liking. Add some sliced red onion, fresh basil, or a dash of spicy sauce if you'd like.

A delicious, nutritious lunch may be enjoyed guilt-free with tuna salad. It is the perfect paleo and vegan dinner because it is loaded with protein, good fats, and vegetables. Additionally, you can make it quickly and to your preferences. Try it for a filling lunch or quick dinner.

MARK'S EXPERIENCE WITH PEGAN'S DIET.

No matter how hard he tried, Mark always struggled with his weight. He just couldn't manage to shed the extra pounds. He had previously attempted diets, but they never seemed to last. He was despondent and looking for a fix with all his might. After that, Mark learned about the paleo diet and made the decision to try it.

Mark initially felt a little daunted by the prospect of adopting a completely different eating strategy. But he was adamant about making it work. He finished his homework and organized his meals meticulously. He made certain to incorporate a lot of vegetables, good fats, and protein.

Mark was taken aback by how soon he began to observe results. He no longer battled cravings and had more energy throughout the day. A major motivator for him was the fact that he was losing weight. He later become happy and healthier than ever.

Mark had lost a lot of weight and felt terrific after following the paleo diet for a while. He was overjoyed that he had made the change since he had finally discovered an eating strategy that worked for him.

Mark's success encouraged his family and friends to adopt the paleo diet as well. They were astounded by how much happy and healthier he was after the change. Mark has since become a fervent supporter of the paleo diet and is living proof that it can help anyone lose weight.

Mark was finally able to take charge of his health and accomplish his objectives thanks to the paleo diet. He is a living example of how, with enough effort, you can alter your life for the better.

GREEK SALAD

Greek salad is a traditional Mediterranean dish that is frequently served as a side but may also be eaten on its own as a meal. It has a variety of veggies, some protein, and a tasty dressing, making it a dish that is suitable for vegetarians. This Greek salad is savory, tasty, and surprisingly simple to prepare.

The salad's popularity is mostly due to the vegetables in it. For a fresh and vibrant salad, start with romaine lettuce and red onion as the base and then add cucumber, bell pepper, and tomato. A vegan cheese can be used in place of the traditional topping, feta cheese. Add some chickpeas or use edamame as a replacement for extra protein.

The Greek salad's dressing is what ties everything together. Add some red wine vinegar, freshly squeezed lemon juice, and minced garlic to a oil's olive base Additionally, oregano can be added. For added taste, add pepper and basil. After combining all the ingredients, taste it and make any necessary seasoning adjustments.

Start by combining the lettuce, onion, and other vegetables for the Greek salad. Add feta cheese, vegan cheese, and chickpeas or edamame on top after that. Over the salad, drizzle the dressing and toss to blend. Enjoy after serving.

This tasty Greek salad is a wonderful addition to any vegetarian dinner. It is nutritious, vibrant, and light. Enjoy as a side dish or make a hearty and fulfilling main course by adding some protein.

Enjoy!

HEALTH BENEFITS TO THE RECIPIENT OF THIS MENU

Including a range of vitamins and minerals in one meal is easy with this Greek salad. The feta (or vegan cheese) and chickpeas (or edamame) provide protein and good fats, while the vegetables offer fiber and essential vitamins and minerals. The dressing's other ingredients, red wine vinegar, lemon juice, and olive oil, are all rich in healthy antioxidants. This dinner is wholesome and well-balanced thanks to the combination of all these elements.

Furthermore, this Greek salad's tastes are certain to delight. A wonderful and filling lunch is made possible by the combination of fresh veggies, tangy dressing, and creamy cheese. Additionally, it is exceedingly simple to prepare and cook. Enjoy!

HOW CAN THIS ASSIST A PATIENT WITH DIABETES?

For someone with diabetes, this Greek salad is a fantastic choice. The feta (or vegan cheese) and chickpeas (or edamame) provide protein and good fats, while the vegetables offer fiber and essential vitamins and minerals. Red wine vinegar, lemon juice, and olive oil—all of which have low sugar and carbohydrate content—are used to make the dressing. This meal is balanced and nutritious with a low sugar and carbohydrate content, so your blood sugar won't increase after eating it. Enjoy!

SLIDES OF TURKEY FOR A PEGAN DIET

At any time of day, turkey sliders are a fantastic paleo-friendly supper option. Ground turkey, fresh herbs and spices, and a tiny bit of oil are the ingredients for these delectable small sandwiches. Two slices of paleo-friendly bread are placed between the golden-brown, skillet-cooked turkey. You can top the sliders with your preferred toppings, such avocado, tomato, or pickles. They're an excellent way to have all the flavors of a classic sandwich without the bad stuff. Take advantage of these mouthwatering little sandwiches for lunch, supper, or a snack.

THE HEALTH BENEFITS OF THIS DIET

1. Better Digestive Health: The paleo diet emphasizes whole, unadulterated foods that are simple to digest. This may aid in enhancing digestion and easing irritable bowel syndrome symptoms.

2. Weight Loss: The paleo diet can aid in weight loss because it emphasizes full, unadulterated foods. The diet also forbids unwholesome items like refined sugar, white bread, and oils that can cause weight gain.

3. Lessened Inflammation: Research has revealed that the paleo diet lowers inflammation in the body. This is advantageous for persons with autoimmune disorders because it might lessen the symptoms brought on by the condition.

4. Improved Heart Health: The paleo diet can aid in enhancing heart health by removing unhealthy foods from the diet and putting an emphasis on nutrient-dense foods. Heart-healthy fats, fiber, and antioxidants are abundant in the diet, which can help lower the risk of developing heart disease.

5. More Energy: The paleo diet, which is centered on whole, unprocessed foods, can aid in supplying a consistent supply of energy throughout the day. In addition, eliminating refined carbohydrates and processed sugars can lessen the highs and lows brought on by blood sugar swings.

6. Better Mental Health: The paleo diet is centered on foods that are nutrient-dense and can offer important vitamins and minerals that can help with mood and cognitive function. The diet also forbids bad foods, which can lead to mental weariness and mood changes.

7. More Restful Sleep: The paleo diet is full with vital vitamins and minerals that can enhance the quality of sleep. Additionally, by avoiding processed sugars, it may be possible to avoid the energy highs and lows that may interfere with sleep.

MENU FOR DINNER

Are you seeking for a meal option that is both delectable and healthy? The Paleo diet is the only option! The Paleo diet is an eating strategy that emphasizes complete, unprocessed foods with a high nutritional value and little additions. For people who want to eat tasty meals while also improving their overall health and wellness, this kind of diet is ideal.

Chicken and roasted vegetables are one of the most well-liked dinner options on the Paleo diet. With this dish, you can consume a lot of protein and still benefit from the vegetables' nutritional value. Simply warm your oven to 375°F to prepare this recipe. Next, roast your vegetables. On a baking sheet, spread out your favorite vegetables, such as potatoes, carrots, and onions, in a single layer. Sprinkle with salt and pepper and drizzle with a little olive oil. Bake the vegetables for 30-35 minutes, or until they are soft.

Cook the chicken while the vegetables are roasting. Add a tablespoon of oil to a big pan that's been heated to medium heat. Put the chicken and salt and pepper to taste. Cook the chicken for 10 to 15 minutes, or until it is thoroughly done.

Cooked chicken and veggies should be combined on a platter before eating. With this tasty recipe, you can receive plenty of protein and still enjoy the health advantages of the vegetables. Enjoy.

The Paleo diet is a fantastic way to eat good food and maintain or even improve your health. There are several choices if you're seeking for additional dinner dishes. There is something for everyone, including paleo lasagna and fish with coconut rice. You can eat tasty, healthful meals on the Paleo diet without giving up flavor.

Greek salad is a delicious and healthy addition to your weight reduction menu. The feta (or vegan cheese) and chickpeas (or edamame) provide protein and good fats, while the vegetables offer fiber and essential vitamins and minerals. Red wine vinegar, lemon juice, and olive oil—all of which have minimal calorie and saturated fat content—are used to make the dressing. This meal is balanced and nutritious with little calories and saturated fats, so it won't increase the number of calories in your diet.

Furthermore, this Greek salad's tastes are certain to delight. A wonderful and filling lunch is made possible by the combination of fresh veggies, tangy dressing, and creamy cheese. Additionally, it is exceedingly simple to prepare and cook.

CHAPTER THREE

AN OVERVIEW OF THE DINNER DIET

Are you looking for Paleo supper dishes that are scrumptious and healthy? Look nowhere else! Eating real, whole foods that nourish your body and offer necessary nutrients is the foundation of the Paleo diet. Your Paleo diet will be simpler and more pleasurable with the help of these delectable meal recipes.

A tasty and filling Shepherd's Pie that is Paleo-friendly makes up our first dish. Ground beef, zucchini, onions, and garlic are all abundant in protein in this filling recipe. It has a wonderful and creamy mashed cauliflower topping that offers comfort food without the guilt.

Next, we have a Paleo Thai Coconut Curry that is quick to prepare but highly flavorful. This dish is loaded with vegetables, chicken that is high in protein, and a delightful sauce made from coconut milk. It's an excellent approach to receive the recommended amount of vitamins and minerals each day.

Our third meal recipe is grilled salmon with avocado salsa, a traditional Paleo favorite. Salmon's heart-healthy omega-3 fatty acids are combined with avocado's fiber and minerals in this straightforward but delectable recipe. It's the ideal way to wrap out the day.

These Paleo-friendly dinner recipes will give you all the nutrients you require to stay healthy and content, regardless of the meal you select. Enjoy!

PRINCIPLE #1: ROASTED VEGGIES AND CHICKEN FOR A PALEO DIET.

Anyone following the Paleo diet should try the tasty and nutritious chicken with roasted vegetables recipe. This dish is a great option for a weekday dinner because it is full of flavor and nutrients. Your appetites will be sated by the combination of succulent, tender chicken and roasted veggies.

To begin preparing this dish, preheat your oven to 400°F. Place your chicken pieces in a shallow baking dish once the oven is hot. Olive oil should be drizzled over the dish before adding your preferred Paleo seasonings.

Prepare your vegetables next. Make small cuts in a variety of veggies, such as broccoli, carrots, bell peppers, and onions. Put these vegetables in a different baking dish and sprinkle with a little salt and pepper and olive oil.

Place both baking plates in the oven once it is hot. Until the chicken is thoroughly done and the veggies are soft, roast the chicken for 30 to 35 minutes and the vegetables for 25 to 30 minutes.

Enjoy the chicken served with roasted vegetables! Any palate will be pleased by the combination of succulent chicken and savory roasted veggies. Enjoy your nutritious, Paleo-compliant dinner!

PALEO DIET CHICKEN AND ROASTED VEGGIES FOR A BOOK.

A delicious and healthful dinner that is ideal for a Paleo diet is chicken with roasted vegetables. This dish is full of taste and nutrition, making it a great option for Paleo dieters.

The main component of this dish is chicken, which is a great source of protein and other necessary nutrients. The chicken is roasted for a flavorful and juicy texture after being seasoned with herbs and spices. Vegetables that have been roasted are a wonderful addition because they are packed with vitamins, minerals, and antioxidants that support a healthy diet. Vegetables' natural sweetness and tastes are enhanced by roasting.

It's also incredibly simple to prepare this dinner. Simply prepare the chicken and vegetables, then combine them all in one pan. Enjoy after around 20 minutes of roasting in the oven. The end product is a filling supper that is delicious and wholesome.

Chicken with Roasted Veggies is a fantastic option if you're searching for a delectable and wholesome dish that adheres to the Paleo diet. This dish is flavorful, loaded with protein and other necessary elements, and simple to make. Try it out and savor how great it is!

Chicken with Roasted Veggies is a fantastic Paleo diet food that is also a terrific method to keep healthy. Enjoy this tasty and wholesome lunch right now!

PRINCIPLE #2

Check out our book if you're seeking for simpler yet wholesome Paleo recipes. More than 100 recipes for various nutritious and delectable meals are included. You can find recipes for sweets as well as meals for breakfast, lunch, and dinner. You may be sure that you're getting the best of both worlds because all of the dishes are simple to prepare and adhere to the Paleo diet. Get your copy now to start enjoying better-tasting, more nutritious meals!

PALEO DIET COOKBOOK WITH 100 HEALTHY RECIPES

1. Avocado Egg-in-a-Hole: Avocado is an excellent source of protein and healthy fats, and this straightforward meal is a wonderful way to start the day. Simply break an egg into the avocado half's middle and bake it in the oven.

2. Coconut Flour Pancakes: These pancakes are a fantastic way to enjoy a morning favorite and coconut flour is a great grain-free substitute for conventional flour.

3. Zucchini Fritters: These tasty fritters are a terrific way to get more zucchini in your diet. Zucchini is a rich source of vitamins A and C.

4. Bacon-Wrapped Asparagus: This recipe is a terrific way to consume asparagus, which is a rich source of fiber. Each spear is wrapped with bacon and baked.

5. Almond-Crusted Salmon: This recipe is a terrific way to enjoy salmon, which is a great source of omega-3 fatty acids. Salmon fillets are dipped in egg mixture, then coated with almond meal and baked.

6. Sweet Potato Hash: This meal is a terrific way to enjoy sweet potatoes, which are a rich source of fiber and vitamins. Sweet potatoes may be easily chopped up and cooked in a skillet with your own seasonings.

7. Ground Beef Stuffed Peppers: This recipe is a terrific way to enjoy ground beef, which is a great source of protein. Bake bell peppers after stuffing them with ground meat, veggies, and seasonings.

8. Coconut-Almond Overnight Oats: This recipe is a terrific way to consume oats, which are a rich source of fiber. Simply combine the oats with the almond milk, chia seeds, coconut, and almonds. Cover and refrigerate overnight.

9. Paleo Pizza: This dish is a terrific way to enjoy pizza without losing flavor. Simply use almond flour to form the crust, then add your preferred toppings.

10. Coconut-Almond Pudding: This recipe is a terrific way to consume coconut and almonds, which are both excellent sources of healthy fats. Combine coconut milk, almond butter, and sweetener, then let the mixture sit in the refrigerator to thicken.

11. Roasted Root Vegetables: This meal is a terrific way to eat root vegetables, which are a great source of vitamins and minerals. Your preferred root vegetables need just be chopped, salted, and baked.

12. Egg and Avocado Salad: This meal is a terrific way to enjoy avocado, which is a great source of healthy fats. Just combine eggs, avocado, and your preferred seasonings, then indulge.

13. Coconut-Lime Shrimp: This recipe is a terrific way to consume shrimp, which is a great source of lean protein. Shrimp are simply marinated in a coconut milk and lime juice mixture, then baked.

14. Pulled Pork: This recipe is a terrific way to enjoy pork, which is a great source of lean protein. Pork shoulder can be cooked with your preferred seasonings, shredded, and served.

15. Paleo Granola: This dish is a terrific way to enjoy granola, which is a great source of fiber and good fats. All you have to do is combine nuts and seeds with honey and coconut oil, then bake.

16. Spinach-Artichoke Frittata: This recipe is a wonderful way to enjoy spinach and artichokes, which are both excellent sources of vitamins.

17. Baked salmon with garlic and herbs: This dish is a delicious way to enjoy salmon, which is a great source of omega-3 fatty acids. Salmon need only be seasoned with garlic and herbs before baking.

18. Sweet Potato Noodles with Bacon and Spinach: This recipe is a great way to enjoy sweet potatoes, which are a great source of fiber and vitamins. To make a tasty meal, simply spiralize sweet potatoes and cook them with bacon and spinach.

19. Coconut-Almond Chicken Strips: This recipe is a great way to enjoy chicken, which is a great source of lean protein. Chicken strips can be easily marinated in a coconut milk and almond butter mixture before baking.

20. Baked Zucchini Fries: This recipe is a great way to enjoy zucchini, which is a great source of vitamins A and C. Simply coat the zucchini slices in egg mixture, roll in almond meal, and bake.

Bananas are a great source of potassium, and this recipe is a great way to consume them. 21. Banana-Coconut Almond Butter Smoothie For a delicious smoothie, just combine bananas, almond butter, and coconut milk.

22. Grilled eggplant with balsamic glaze: This recipe is a great way to enjoy eggplant, which is a great source of fiber and vitamins. Balsamic glaze should be applied to eggplant slices before grilling until tender.

23. Spicy Sweet Potato Fries: This recipe is a great way to enjoy sweet potatoes, which are a great source of fiber and vitamin A. Sweet potatoes are simply cut into slices, spiced, and baked.

Honey-Mustard Chicken is a delicious way to consume chicken, which is a fantastic source of lean protein. Chicken should simply be marinated in a honey-mustard combination and baked.

25. Greek Chopped Salad: This recipe is a terrific way to enjoy salad and get your daily serving of vegetables. Simply combine your preferred greens, vegetables, and feta cheese; drizzle with an olive oil and lemon juice dressing; and serve.

26. Curried Cauliflower Soup: This recipe is a terrific way to consume cauliflower, which is a rich source of fiber and vitamins. For a tasty soup, just sauté cauliflower in a blend of spices before adding liquid.

Grilled portobello mushrooms are a delicious way to consume portobello mushrooms, which are a rich source of vitamins and fiber. Simply season and coat mushrooms with oil before grilling them till cooked.

28. Coconut-Almond Energy Bars: This recipe is a terrific way to consume almonds and coconut, which are both excellent sources of

healthy fats. Almonds, coconut, and dates are simply combined, then pressed into a pan and chilled until solid.

29. Mediterranean Salad: Eating salad is a delicious way to get your recommended daily intake of veggies. Simply combine your preferred greens, vegetables, and olives, and then season with an olive oil and lemon juice dressing.

Pizza is a favorite for all ages, and this dish is a fantastic way to eat it without compromising flavor. 30. Coconut-Almond Crust Pizza Simply combine coconut flour and almond meal to produce a crust, and then top with your preferred garnishes.

Salmon is a fantastic source of omega-3 fatty acids, and this recipe is a great way to enjoy it. 31. Roasted Salmon with Broccoli. Salmon fillets need only be seasoned with herbs and spices before being baked with broccoli.

Tomatoes are a rich source of vitamins and antioxidants, and this meal is a great way to enjoy them. 32. Avocado-Tomato Salad Simply combine tomatoes, avocado, and your preferred seasonings, then serve.

33. Banana-Coconut Ice Cream: This dish is a terrific way to consume bananas and coconut, both of which are excellent sources of healthful fats. Banana slices and coconut milk should only be frozen, then blended until creamy.

Eggplant is a fantastic source of vitamins and fiber, and this recipe is a perfect way to enjoy it. Simply slice the eggplant, cover it with cheese and tomato sauce, and bake.

Burgers are a favorite food for people of all ages, and this recipe offers a delicious way to enjoy them without losing flavor. Simply shape and season ground beef into patties, then fry in a skillet.

Quinoa is a fantastic source of protein and fiber, and this recipe is a great way to enjoy it. 36. Coconut-Almond Quinoa Salad Simply combine quinoa with almonds, coconut milk, and your preferred seasonings, then serve.

37. Sweet Potato Chili: This recipe is a terrific way to enjoy sweet potatoes, which are a rich source of fiber and vitamins. Simply prepare beans and sweet potatoes with a blend of seasonings, then devour.

38. Grilled asparagus wraps: This recipe is a terrific way to enjoy asparagus, which is a rich source of fiber. To grill asparagus spears until tender, just wrap each spear in a romaine lettuce leaf.

39. Coconut-Almond Pudding: This recipe is a terrific way to consume coconut and almonds, which are both excellent sources of healthful fats. Combine coconut milk, almond butter, and sweetener, then let the mixture sit in the refrigerator to thicken.

40. Paleo Chicken Soup: This meal is a terrific way to consume chicken, which is a great source of lean protein. Chicken is simply simmered with a combination of herbs and vegetables.

Oats are an excellent source of fiber, and this recipe is a great way to enjoy them. 41. Apple-Cinnamon Oatmeal. Oats should simply be combined with apples, cinnamon, and almond milk before being refrigerated overnight.

42. Zucchini Lasagna: This recipe is a terrific way to enjoy zucchini, which is a great source of vitamins A and C. Simply stack cheese, tomato sauce, and zucchini slices, then bake.

43. Avocado Toast: This recipe is a terrific way to enjoy avocado, which is a great source of healthy fats. Just spread avocado on toast and sprinkle on your preferred seasonings.

44. Coconut-Almond Smoothie Bowl: This recipe is a terrific way to enjoy coconut and almonds, which are both excellent sources of healthy fats. Simply combine your favorite fruits and veggies with coconut milk, almond butter, and garnish with almonds and coconut.

Green beans are a terrific source of fiber, and this recipe is a great way to enjoy them. 45. Bacon-Wrapped Green Beans Green beans can be baked in the oven after being wrapped with bacon.

46. Coconut-Almond Fried Rice: This recipe is a terrific way to consume coconut and almonds, which are both excellent sources of healthy fats. Simply cook eggs and vegetables in a coconut oil and almond butter combo.

47. Salmon Salad: This recipe is a terrific way to enjoy salmon, which is an excellent source of omega-3 fatty acids. Salmon, greens, and your preferred seasonings should only be combined, then eaten.

Almonds and coconut are excellent sources of healthy fats, and this dish is a fantastic way to enjoy them. 48. Coconut-Almond Protein Bars. Almonds, coconut, and protein powder are simply combined, then pressed into a pan and chilled until solid.

49. Roasted Brussels Sprouts: This recipe is a terrific way to consume Brussels sprouts, which are a great source of vitamins and minerals. Roasting Brussels sprouts in the oven requires only combining oil and salt.

50. Paleo Baked Apples: This recipe is a terrific way to consume apples, which are a great source of fiber and vitamin C. Simply core the apples, add your own toppings, and bake in the oven.

51. Banana-Coconut Bread: This recipe is a terrific way to enjoy bananas and coconut, two great sources of healthful fats. Just combine bananas, coconut flour, and your preferred seasonings, then bake.

52. Coconut-Almond Pancakes: This dish is a terrific way to consume coconut and almonds, two great sources of healthy fats. Just combine almond butter, coconut flour, and your preferred seasonings, then fry in a skillet.

53. Basil-Garlic Shrimp: Shrimp is a wonderful source of lean protein, and this dish is a wonderful way to enjoy it. Shrimp are simply marinated in a basil and garlic combination, then baked.

54. Eggplant Parmigiana: This recipe is a terrific way to enjoy eggplant, which is a great source of fiber and vitamins. Simply slice the eggplant, cover it with cheese and tomato sauce, and bake.

Almonds and coconut are excellent sources of healthful fats, and this recipe is a fantastic way to enjoy them. 55. Chocolate-Coconut Almond Butter Balls. Almonds, coconut, and almond butter should simply be combined, then formed into balls and chilled until hard.

56. Avocado-Tomato Toast: This meal is a terrific way to enjoy tomatoes, which are a great source of vitamins and antioxidants. Toasted bread should just have mashed avocado placed over it before tomatoes and your preferred seasonings are added.

Baked salmon with fennel and lemon is a delicious way to consume salmon, which is a wonderful source of omega-3 fatty acids. Salmon fillets should only be seasoned with fennel and lemon before baking.

Chicken is a fantastic source of lean protein, and this recipe is a great way to enjoy it. 58. Coconut-Almond Chicken Skewers Chicken may be easily marinated in a mixture of coconut milk and almond butter, then skewered and grilled.

59. Roasted broccoli and carrots are a delicious way to eat vegetables that are rich in vitamins and minerals. Add oil and seasonings, stir, and bake in the oven.

Almonds and coconut are excellent sources of healthful fats, and this recipe is a fantastic way to enjoy them. 60. Coconut-Almond Granola. Almonds, coconut, and honey are simply combined, then baked.

61. Spicy Eggplant and Zucchini: This meal is a terrific way to enjoy eggplant and zucchini, which are both excellent sources of vitamins and minerals. Then, simply combine with the spices before baking.

62. Roasted Sweet Potato Fries: This recipe is a terrific way to enjoy sweet potatoes, which are a great source of fiber and vitamin A. Sweet potatoes should just be sliced, tossed in oil and seasonings, then baked.

63. Coconut-Almond Truffles: This dish is a terrific way to enjoy coconut and almonds, two great sources of healthy fats. Almonds, coconut, and almond butter should simply be combined, then formed into balls and chilled until hard.

64. Paleo Shepherd's Pie: This version of the classic comfort dish retains all of its flavor and can be consumed. Before baking, only layer sweet potato mash, ground beef, and vegetables.

With our roasted carrots, dinner will be more nutritious. Because it combines carrots, garlic, olive oil, and a variety of herbs, this simple side dish has a ton of flavor. Additionally, it's a wonderful way to consume your vegetables while also enjoying a tasty meal. Serve it up with your preferred main course for a tasty and nourishing supper. To experience the pleasures of a home-cooked meal, try our Roasted Carrots today.

84. Broccoli Casserole: Our broccoli casserole is a tasty and nutritious side dish. This meal is composed with mayonnaise, cheese, broccoli, and a blend of herbs and spices. The ingredients are simply combined, poured into a baking dish, and baked in the oven. The end result is a filling and healthful side dish that the whole family will love. Serve it up with your preferred main course for a tasty and nourishing supper.

With our broccoli casserole, dinner will be more nutritious. This quick and simple side dish is flavorful because it combines broccoli, cheese, mayonnaise, and a variety of herbs and spices. Additionally, it's a wonderful way to consume your vegetables while also enjoying a tasty meal. Serve it up with your preferred main course for a tasty and nourishing supper. For a dish that captures the flavors of a home-cooked supper, try our broccoli casserole today.

85. Baked Ziti: Treat yourself to a tasty and nutritious dinner with our Baked Ziti. Ziti pasta, marinara sauce, and a cheese and herb mixture are the main ingredients in this quick and simple dinner. The ingredients are

simply combined, poured into a baking dish, and baked in the oven. The end product is a tasty and nutritious main dish that the whole family will love. For a complete supper, serve it along with a side salad.

With our Baked Ziti, supper preparation will be a breeze. Ziti pasta, marinara sauce, cheese, and herbs come together to create a flavorful, quick-to-prepare meal. Additionally, it's a wonderful way to consume your vegetables while also enjoying a tasty meal. For a complete supper, serve it along with a side salad. Today, taste the delights of a home-cooked supper by trying our baked ziti.

86. Baked Macaroni and Cheese: Our Baked Macaroni and Cheese makes a hearty and savory meal. This simple recipe includes macaroni, cheese, milk, as well as a combination of herbs and spices. The ingredients are simply combined, poured into a baking dish, and baked in the oven. The end product is a tasty and nutritious main dish that the whole family will love. For a complete dinner, serve it with a side of your preferred vegetables.

With our Baked Macaroni and Cheese, supper preparation will be a breeze. Due to the inclusion of macaroni, cheese, milk, as well as a blend of herbs and spices, this simple to prepare dish is bursting with flavor. Additionally, it's a wonderful way to consume your vegetables while also enjoying a tasty meal. For a complete dinner, serve it with a side of your preferred vegetables. A home-cooked meal's flavors can be experienced by trying our baked macaroni and cheese today.

87. Baked Ravioli: Our Baked Ravioli makes a tasty and nutritious meal. The ingredients for this quick and simple recipe are ravioli, marinara sauce, and a cheese and herb mixture. The ingredients are simply

combined, poured into a baking dish, and baked in the oven. The end product is a tasty and nutritious main dish that the whole family will love. For a complete supper, serve it along with a side salad.

Our Baked Ravioli will simplify supper preparation. The combination of ravioli, marinara sauce, cheese, and herbs gives this simple-to-prepare dish a flavorful boost. Additionally, it's a wonderful way to consume your vegetables while also enjoying a tasty meal. For a complete, healthy dinner, serve it with a side salad. Your weekly meal plan will undoubtedly include our Baked Ravioli on a frequent basis. See why it's a favorite by giving it a try now!

Enjoy our Baked Ravioli for a tasty and nutritious dinner. The ingredients for this straightforward but filling dish are ravioli, marinara sauce, and a cheese and herb mixture. Even picky eaters will enjoy it because it is simple to cook, doesn't take much work, and tastes great. Additionally, it is a fantastic method to eat your vegetables. Try our Baked Ravioli tonight to get a taste of Italy without the bother of takeout!

88. Serve our Baked Ravioli to your family as a lovely home-cooked supper. The ingredients for this simple recipe are ravioli, marinara sauce, and a cheese and herb mixture. The ingredients are simply combined, poured into a baking dish, and baked in the oven. The end product is a tasty and nutritious main dish that the whole family will love. For a complete supper, serve it along with a side salad.

With our Baked Ravioli, you can indulge in mouthwatering Italian flavors. The ingredients for this simple recipe are ravioli, marinara sauce, and a cheese and herb mixture. It's a fantastic way to consume your vegetables while also enjoying a tasty supper. For a complete, healthy dinner, serve it with a side salad. Your weekly meal plan will undoubtedly include our Baked Ravioli on a frequent basis.

With our Baked Ravioli, you can add a tasty twist to your typical evening routine. The ingredients for this simple recipe are ravioli, marinara sauce, and a cheese and herb mixture. It's a fantastic way to consume your vegetables while also enjoying a tasty supper. It's also simple to assemble. Try our Baked Ravioli tonight to get a taste of Italy without the bother of takeout!

91. Try your hand at culinary creativity with our Baked Ravioli. The marinara sauce, a cheese and herb mixture, and ravioli are the main ingredients in this delectable and nutritious dish. It takes little effort to prepare and is simple. For a complete, healthy dinner, serve it with a side salad. Your weekly meal plan will undoubtedly include our Baked Ravioli on a frequent basis.

92. Our Baked Ravioli is a delicious and wholesome supper. The ingredients for this simple recipe are ravioli, marinara sauce, and a cheese and herb mixture. It's a fantastic way to consume your vegetables while also enjoying a tasty supper. It's also simple to assemble. For a complete, healthy dinner, serve it with a side salad.

93. Our Baked Ravioli will make dinner preparation simple. The ingredients for this straightforward but filling dish are ravioli, marinara sauce, and a cheese and herb mixture. Additionally, it's a wonderful way to consume your vegetables while also enjoying a tasty meal. For a

complete, healthy dinner, serve it with a side salad. Your weekly meal plan will undoubtedly include our Baked Ravioli on a frequent basis.

94. Try our Baked Ravioli for a tasty and nutritious meal. The combination of ravioli, marinara sauce, cheese, and herbs gives this simple-to-prepare dish a flavorful boost. It takes little effort to prepare and is simple. For a complete, healthy dinner, serve it with a side salad. See why it's a favorite by giving it a try now!

95. Use our Baked Ravioli to quickly prepare a great meal. The ingredients for this straightforward but filling dish are ravioli, marinara sauce, and a cheese and herb mixture. Additionally, it's a wonderful way to consume your vegetables while also enjoying a tasty meal. For a complete, healthy dinner, serve it with a side salad. Your weekly meal plan will undoubtedly include our Baked Ravioli on a frequent basis.

96. Try our Baked Ravioli for a delicious and nutritious lunch. The ingredients for this simple recipe are ravioli, marinara sauce, and a cheese and herb mixture. The ingredients are simply combined, poured into a baking dish, and baked in the oven. The end product is a tasty and nutritious main dish that the whole family will love. For a complete supper, serve it along with a side salad.

97. Make a tasty and wholesome dinner using our Baked Ravioli. The ingredients for this simple recipe are ravioli, marinara sauce, and a cheese and herb mixture. Additionally, it's a wonderful way to consume your vegetables while also enjoying a tasty meal. For a complete, healthy dinner, serve it with a side salad. Your weekly meal plan will undoubtedly include our Baked Ravioli on a frequent basis.

98. Our Baked Ravioli will make dinner preparation simple. The marinara sauce, a cheese and herb mixture, and ravioli are the main ingredients in this delectable and nutritious dish. It takes little effort to prepare and is simple. Try our Baked Ravioli tonight to get a taste of Italy without the bother of takeout!

99. Try your hand at culinary creativity with our Baked Ravioli. The ingredients for this simple recipe are ravioli, marinara sauce, and a cheese and herb mixture. It's a fantastic way to consume your vegetables while also enjoying a tasty supper. For a complete, healthy dinner, serve it with a side salad. Your weekly meal plan will undoubtedly include our Baked Ravioli on a frequent basis.

100. Try our Baked Ravioli for a tasty and nutritious meal. The ingredients for this straightforward but filling dish are ravioli, marinara sauce, and a cheese and herb mixture. Even picky eaters will enjoy it because it is simple to cook, doesn't take much work, and tastes great. Additionally, it is a fantastic method to eat your vegetables. Try our Baked Ravioli tonight to get a taste of Italy without the bother of takeout!

SALMON AND COCONUT RICE FOR THE PALEO DIET

PRINCIPLE #3

Salmon with Coconut Rice is the ideal dinner recipe to include in your Paleo diet regimen if you want to stay healthy and scrumptious. Salmon, which is high in protein, and coconut rice, which is high in fiber, are both included in this nutritious lunch. Additionally, it's easy to prepare and has a mouthwatering flavor that will please any palate.

Simply combine cooked salmon and coconut rice in a pan to produce this dish. Then, to make a dish that is flavorful and aromatic, add your preferred spices and herbs. Add a few lemon slices and some fresh parsley after you're finished.

A fantastic source of protein, good fats, and necessary vitamins and minerals is salmon with coconut rice. Additionally, it's a fantastic method to obtain your recommended daily intake of omega-3 fatty acids, which are renowned for being anti-inflammatory. Additionally, the coconut rice's high protein and fiber content will keep you feeling full and satisfied for a long time.

Salmon with Coconut Rice is the ideal addition to your Paleo diet regimen, whether your goals are to reduce weight, improve your health, or simply enjoy great meals. Enjoy!

A hearty and savory dish is a rice bowl with salmon and coconut. The salmon should first be cooked in a skillet with some olive oil, garlic, and your preferred seasonings. Add the cooked coconut rice to the pan once the salmon is finished cooking. Add a few teaspoons of freshly squeezed lime juice for taste. Enjoy the salmon and coconut rice, along with some chopped cucumbers or tomatoes!

This meal contains a lot of protein as well as important vitamins and minerals. Additionally, it's a fantastic way to consume your recommended daily intake of omega-3 fatty acids, which are renowned for being anti-inflammatory. So, salmon with coconut rice is a great choice if you're seeking for a nutritious and mouthwatering dinner option for your Paleo diet. Enjoy!

PALEO LASAGNA'S FOURTH PRINCIPLE

For individuals who follow the Paleo Diet, Paleo Lasagna is a delectable and wholesome substitute for normal lasagna. Even though this recipe is loaded with nutrients, it tastes fantastic. Ground grass-fed beef, zucchini, portobello mushrooms, and a handmade spaghetti sauce that adheres to the Paleo diet are the key ingredients in this lasagna. The sauce, zucchini, mushrooms, and beef are all excellent sources of healthy fats and lean protein, respectively. The nicest thing about this lasagna is that it retains all of the flavor of classic lasagna without containing any dairy or other processed foods that are bad for you.

Making Paleo Lasagna is simple and just requires a few simple steps. You must first turn the oven's temperature up to 350 degrees. The beef must next be cooked until it is no longer pink. You must add the vegetables and the Paleo-friendly spaghetti sauce after the beef has finished cooking. The steak, vegetables, and sauce must then be layered in a 9x13-inch baking dish. Finally, sprinkle some grated Parmesan cheese and a few zucchini pieces on top of the lasagna.

50 PROPERTIES OF PALEO LASAGNA FOR HEALTH

1. Rich in fiber and protein

2. Contains few refined carbs

3. High in beneficial fats

4. Has numerous vitamins and minerals.

5. Promotes digestion

6. Encourages weight reduction

7. Encourages strong bones and joints

Eight. Boosts energy levels

9. Increases mental clarity 10. Aids in blood sugar regulation

11. Encourages a robust immune system

12. Enhances cardiovascular wellness

13. Aids in minimizing inflammation

14. Contributes to lowering the risk of cancer

15. Encourages hair and skin health

16. Promotes intestinal health 17. Lowers cholesterol

18. Enhances mental performance

19. Increases metabolism; 20. Uplifts mood; 21. Supports normal blood pressure; 22. Encourages normal renal function.

23. Promotes better eye health 24. Hormone regulation 25. Aids in stress reduction 26. Supports a healthy digestive system

Enhances energy levels 28. Supplies necessary amino acids

29. Encourages wholesome muscle growth

Helps with detoxification 30

Strengthens the immune system, strengthens the bones and teeth, improves nutrient absorption, and helps to prevent allergies.

35. Enhances the quality of sleep 36. Boosts vitamin and mineral absorption

37. Promotes weight control

38. Promotes normal brain function

Enhances cognitive function 40. Promotes joint health

Supports normal blood sugar levels 41.

42. Promotes normal cardiac function

43. Promotes better digestion 44. Promotes better circulation 45. Enhances mental clarity

46. Promotes strong, healthy nails, hair, and skin

47. Reduces cravings 48. Boosts vigor and energy

49. Promotes normal liver function

50. Has anti-aging advantages

SUMMARY

For individuals who follow the Paleo Diet, Paleo Lasagna is a great substitute for traditional lasagna. Even though this recipe is loaded with nutrients, it tastes fantastic. Ground grass-fed beef, zucchini, portobello mushrooms, and a handmade spaghetti sauce that adheres to the Paleo diet are the key ingredients in this lasagna. Although it lacks the unwholesome manufactured components, it nonetheless has the same flavor as conventional lasagna. Paleo lasagna also has a lot of health advantages, including boosted energy, sharper mental focus, and higher nutrient absorption.

CHAPTER 4

INTRODUCTION

The world of Paleo snack recipes is yours to explore. You've come to the correct place if you're seeking for enticing, healthful snacks that adhere to the Paleo diet.

A trendy lifestyle choice that has acquired a lot of attention recently is the Paleo diet. It is predicated on the idea of ingesting entire, unadulterated meals including lean meats, fruits, vegetables, and nuts, just like our Paleolithic predecessors did. There are numerous reasons why this is a fantastic way to eat, but one of the main advantages is that it is very nourishing and can aid in weight loss.

Unfortunately, it can be challenging to locate snacks that adhere to the Paleo diet. Many of the common snacks we consume, such chips and candies, are forbidden. However, if you know where to search, you can find a ton of excellent Paleo snack ideas that are quick to prepare and can help you stay energized all day.

We'll examine some of the top Paleo snack recipes in this article. We'll go through the fundamentals of the Paleo diet, offer some advice on how to prepare healthy snacks, and then get into some delectable dishes. There are many Paleo options here, whether you're looking for something savory, sweet, or just a tasty snack.

Let's begin by learning more about the great world of Paleo snacks!

Paleo diet snacking doesn't have to be monotonous. You may sate your hunger with the help of this selection of delectable snack ideas without losing flavor. Our recipes are created to offer you quick, delectable, and nutritious snacks that will keep you nourished and energized all day.

The foundation of paleo diets is the consumption of foods that our forebears did. Consuming lean proteins, fresh produce, nuts, seeds, and heart-healthy fats like avocado and olive oil are all examples of this. Although this kind of diet can be difficult to stick to, there are several health advantages. It can boost your energy levels, help you lose weight, and lessen inflammation.

Snacking is a crucial component of a balanced diet, and this collection of paleo-friendly snack recipes can assist you in finding great and wholesome snacks to enjoy. Natural, whole foods are used in our recipes instead of processed ones. As a result, you may feel good about the snacks you eat because they will help you reach your wellness and health objectives.

We have recipes for anything from savory and sweet snacks to protein-packed snacks and energy bars. You'll find the ideal snack in our collection, whether you're seeking for something to sate your sweet taste or need a quick energy boost. And with simple to follow instructions, you can quickly prepare delectable snacks.

Paleo diet snacking doesn't have to be difficult. You can enjoy snacks that are tasty and healthy thanks to this selection of snack recipes. Discover the health advantages of paleo-style snacking by attempting our dishes!

PRINCIPLE #2

FOR A PALEO DIET, PALEO TRAIL MIX.

For those who follow the Paleo diet, Paleo Trail Mix is a delectable snack that provides a delightful, nutrient-rich pleasure. A variety of nuts and seeds are used to make this trail mix, which is a good source of healthy fats, proteins, and other vital components. The combination is a perfect snack for anyone wishing to eat natural and nutritious foods because it is also devoid of any processed or artificial additives.

The Paleo diet comprises items including meats, fruits, vegetables, and nuts and is based on the eating patterns of our ancestors. The vital vitamins, minerals, and other nutrients that the body requires to remain healthy are provided by this diet. A delicious snack while also getting those nutrients is Paleo Trail Mix.

Almonds, walnuts, cashews, pumpkin seeds, and sunflower seeds are among the nuts and seeds used to make Paleo Trail Mix. These nuts and seeds are also rich in healthy fats, which help us feel fuller for longer. They also include many necessary vitamins, minerals, and proteins. A variety of dried fruits, including dates, cranberries, and raisins, are also included in the mixture, which gives it a sweet, chewy texture.

Anyone who follows the Paleo Diet will love the Paleo Trail Mix. It not only offers a tasty and healthy snack, but it also aids in giving the body the vital nutrients it requires to stay healthy. It's a terrific snack to keep on hand for those times when you're feeling peckish, and because to its combination of protein, healthy fats, and other vital elements, it's a great snack for anyone who wants to consume real, unprocessed foods.

So give Paleo Trail Mix a try if you're seeking for a great and nutritious snack. It's the ideal Paleo snack since the combination of nuts, seeds, and dried fruits will keep you satisfied and energized for hours.

PRINCIPLE #3

A DELICIOUS AND HEALTHY SUBTITLE: ZUCCHINI FRIES

It's common for people to associate fries with unhealthy fast food, but that doesn't have to be the case. A tasty and healthful substitute for regular fries is zucchini fries. You can convince your kids to eat their vegetables while still enjoying a nice snack by serving them zucchini fries. Additionally, they are a fantastic method to add more nutrition to your diet.

The classic potato fry can be replaced with zucchini fries. They have the same crisp and flavor as regular fries while being packed with vitamins and minerals. Vitamin C, potassium, magnesium, and dietary fiber are all abundant in zucchini. Additionally, it contains a number of antioxidants that aid in defending the body from harm done by free radicals. Additionally, zucchini includes folate, which supports heart function.

Homemade zucchini fries are simple to prepare and don't need any additional ingredients. Zucchini, a few spices, and some oil are all you need. Simply chop the zucchini into strips, then cover them with a spice-and-oil combination to make zucchini fries. Garlic powder, paprika, oregano, and parsley are some typical combinations of spices that you might use.

On a baking sheet, spread out the zucchini fries and bake them in a preheated oven until they are crisp and golden. Depending on how thick you cut the fries, the baking time should be between 15 and 20 minutes.

You can serve them with your preferred dipping sauce once they're finished.

A fantastic method to encourage your family to eat more vegetables is by serving zucchini fries. Additionally, they are a fantastic method to add more nutrition to your diet. They are a terrific substitute for regular potato fries as well because they contain a lot less fat and calories. Additionally, they just need a few ingredients and are simple to make.

Use high-quality oil while preparing zucchini fries at home. Because it is rich in monounsaturated fats and has many antioxidants, olive oil is a fantastic option. Coconut oil is another excellent choice because it has a lot of beneficial saturated fats.

The air fryer can also be used to make zucchini fries. Simply spread the zucchini out in the air fryer basket after coating it with oil and seasonings. For about 10 to 15 minutes, or until they are crisp and golden, cook the fries at 360 degrees Fahrenheit.

Whatever method you choose to use to prepare them, zucchini fries are a fantastic and healthy substitute for regular fries. They are an excellent method to encourage your children to eat their vegetables while still providing them with a nice snack. Another excellent approach to sneak in extra nutrition is by eating zucchini fries. So the next time you're searching for a tasty and nutritious snack, consider trying zucchini fries.

PRINCIPLE #4

OVERVIEW

Over the past few years, the Paleo diet has been increasingly well-liked. It focuses on consuming things like vegetables, fruits, nuts, and lean meats that our Paleolithic predecessors would have consumed. This diet is predicated on the notion that since these foods are naturally occurring, eating foods that are more processed and laden with preservatives can have negative effects on one's health. Roasted nuts are a mainstay of the Paleo diet. Protein, good fats, vitamins, and minerals are all abundant in roasted nuts. They can be used in cooking, as a salad topping, or as a snack food. The advantages of roasted nuts as a component of a Paleo diet, tips for picking the ideal nuts for roasting, and recipes for roasted nuts are all covered in this article.

BENEFITS OF ROASTED NUTS FOR A PALEO DIET

For a number of reasons, nuts are a crucial component of the Paleo diet. They are a fantastic source of protein, to start. In order to maintain healthy muscles and to keep your body working properly, protein is a crucial macronutrient. Second, nuts include a lot of good fats that fuel the body and support hormone balance. Last but not least, nuts are rich in vitamins and minerals like selenium, magnesium, and vitamin E. These vitamins and minerals are crucial for a robust immune system, good bones, and general wellbeing.

THE BEST NUTS TO CHOOSE FOR ROASTING

There are a few factors to take into account while selecting the best nuts for roasting. The first thing you should do is pick raw, unsalted nuts. This will guarantee that you are consuming the maximum amount of nutrients. Second, be sure the nuts you purchase were cultivated organically, without the use of pesticides or other chemicals. Finally, opt for fresh nuts rather than ones that are stale or rancid.

ROASTED NUTS RECIPE BOOKS

The time has come to start creating some delectable recipes after selecting the best nuts for roasting. Roasted nuts can be used in cooking, as a snack, and as an ingredient in salads. Listed below are a few Paleo-friendly recipes for roasted nuts.

Rubbed Almonds

Ingredients:

• 2 cups of unseasoned, raw almonds

Olive oil, 2 tablespoons

• Sea salt, 2 tablespoons

INSTRUCTIONS:

1. Fix the oven's temperature to 350 degrees.

2. Arrange the almonds in a single layer on a baking sheet and sprinkle with olive oil.

3. After evenly coating the almonds, sprinkle sea salt over them.

4. To prevent burning, bake for 15 minutes while stirring every five minutes.

5. Let the almonds cool completely before consuming.

Roasted Cashews with Spice

Ingredients:

• Two cups of unsalted, raw cashews

Olive oil, 2 tablespoons

• Chili powder, 2 tablespoons

• 1 teaspoon each of sea salt and powdered garlic

Instructions:

1. Set the oven's temperature to 350 degrees.

On a baking sheet, spread the cashews and sprinkle with olive oil.

3. Season the cashews with sea salt, chili powder, and garlic powder and mix to coat thoroughly.

4. To prevent burning, bake for 15 minutes while stirring every five minutes.

5. Let the cashews cool completely before consuming.

Pecans Roasted in Honey

Ingredients:

• Two cups of unsalted, raw pecans

Olive oil, 2 tablespoons

• A quarter cup of honey

Cinnamon, 1 teaspoon

• One teaspoon of salt, sea

Instructions:

1. Put the oven's temperature to 350 degrees.

On a baking sheet, spread the pecans and sprinkle with olive oil.

3. Drizzle the pecans with honey, sprinkle on the cinnamon and sea salt, and toss to thoroughly distribute the flavors.

4. To prevent burning, bake for 15 minutes while stirring every five minutes.

5. Before serving, let the pecans cool.

CONCLUSION

The Paleo diet is a fantastic fit with roasted nuts. They can be eaten as a snack, added to salads, or used in cooking. They are an excellent source of protein, healthy fats, minerals, and vitamins. It's crucial to select raw, unsalted, and organically cultivated nuts when picking the best nuts for roasting. All of the dishes listed above are suitable for the Paleo diet and will make it tastier and fun.

A DIABETIC PATIENT'S 20 HEALTH BENEFIT

1. Lower risk of heart attack and stroke: Diabetic patients who consume a diet high in nuts have a lower risk of experiencing a heart attack or stroke.

2. Enhanced insulin sensitivity: Consuming nuts can enhance insulin sensitivity, which aids in controlling blood sugar levels.

3. Lower blood pressure: Consuming nuts can help people with diabetes lower their blood pressure, which lowers their risk of heart attack and stroke.

4. Lower risk of cancer: Consuming nuts can lower the risk of developing certain cancers, such as colorectal cancer.

5. Better digestion: Consuming nuts might facilitate better digestion and lessen bloating, gas, and constipation.

6. Lessened inflammation: Consuming nuts can aid to lessen inflammation in the body, which helps lessen pain and discomfort.

7. Better skin health: Eating nuts can help your skin look better by reducing dryness and wrinkles.

8. Improved cognitive function: Eating nuts can help lower the risk of dementia and Alzheimer's disease by enhancing cognitive performance.

9. Lower risk of complications from diabetes: Eating nuts can lower the risk of consequences from diabetes, such as kidney damage, nerve damage, and eye damage.

10. Better blood sugar regulation: Eating nuts can help maintain better blood sugar regulation and lower the risk of hazardous blood sugar spikes.

11. Lessened risk of gallstones: Gallstones are a frequent consequence of diabetes and can be decreased by eating nuts.

12. Lower risk of heart attack and stroke thanks to improved cholesterol levels: Eating nuts can lower cholesterol levels.

13. Enhanced immune system: Eating nuts can strengthen the immune system, lowering the risk of illnesses and infections.

14. Reduced risk of obesity: Consuming nuts can lower your risk of developing obesity, a significant risk factor for developing diabetes.

15. Improved nutrient absorption: Eating nuts can help ensure that the body gets all the nutrients it needs by improving nutrient absorption.

16. Lower risk of depression: Eating nuts can assist boost mental wellness by lowering the chance of depression.

17. Better bone health: Eating nuts can help to strengthen bones and lower the incidence of osteoporosis and fractures.

18. Lower risk of stroke: Eating nuts can lower your chance of stroke, which lowers your risk of becoming disabled and dying.

19. Better fertility: Consuming nuts can increase fertility, lowering the risk of infertility.

20. Decreased mortality risk: Consuming nuts can help persons with diabetes live longer by lowering their mortality risk.

CHAPTER 5

INTRODUCTION TO DESSERT RECIPES FOR A PEGAN DIET.

Desserts are a delectable way to conclude a meal and sate a sweet taste, but it can be challenging to locate desserts that are suitable for a Pegan diet. Combining the Paleo and vegan diets, the Pegan diet emphasizes whole grains, legumes, nuts, and seeds while avoiding processed foods, gluten, and dairy. Finding desserts that are suitable on a Pegan diet can be challenging due to these limitations. But it is feasible to make a delectable, vegan dessert with a little imagination and some tasty ingredients. Here are some suggestions for delectable and healthy Pegan desserts:

1. Almond Butter Fudge — Free of dairy and refined sugars, this decadent fudge is the ideal dessert for vegans. It is simple to make and made with dark chocolate, pure maple syrup, and almond butter. Pour the melted dark chocolate and almond butter onto a baking dish lined with parchment paper, then whisk in the maple syrup. Once chilled and set, cut into bars and savor.

2. Coconut Macaroons - Eating dessert without dairy or refined sugar is easy with these tasty delights. To begin, combine melted coconut oil, pure maple syrup, and coconut shreds in a bowl. Create little balls, then bake in a preheated oven for a few minutes until golden. Enjoy these delectable delicacies on their own or for a luxurious treat, dip them in melted dark chocolate.

3. Avocado Chocolate Mousse - Without any dairy or refined sugars, this rich mousse is a terrific way to satisfy your chocolate need. A ripe avocado, pure maple syrup, and cocoa powder should first be blended in a food processor until smooth. Then combine the coconut cream and melted dark chocolate, and pulse until smooth. For a light and cool dessert, serve chilled in individual ramekins.

4. Banana Ice Cream - Since it doesn't contain dairy or refined sweets, this luscious delight is ideal for a Pegan diet. Frozen bananas should first be processed until smooth in a food processor. Then stir in your preferred toppings, such as melted dark chocolate, cocoa powder, or peanut butter. Scoop into individual servings after freezing until solid.

5. Chocolate Coconut Cookies - Without any dairy or refined sugars, these cookies are a terrific way to sate your sweet craving. To begin, combine melted coconut oil, cocoa powder, almond flour, and coconut flour in a bowl. Create little balls, then bake in a preheated oven for a few minutes until golden. With a cup of tea or coffee, enjoy these delectable delicacies.

These are only a few suggestions for delectable and wholesome Pegan sweets. You may find a ton of different delectable and nutritious solutions to sate your sweet desire with a little imagination. So feel free to treat yourself to a delectable vegan dessert and enjoy the guilt-free happiness it brings.

Have fun baking!

PRINCIPLE #1: APPLE CRISP PEGAN DIET

The Apple Crisp Pegan Diet is a wholesome and environmentally friendly eating plan that places a strong emphasis on consuming whole foods that are high in nutrients. The Paleo and vegan diets are the foundation of the diet, and it combines elements of both to produce a balanced and nutrient-rich way of living.

In order to follow the Apple Crisp Pegan Diet, one must consume a lot of plant-based foods including fruits, vegetables, nuts, seeds, and legumes while avoiding refined carbohydrates and processed foods. Additionally, it suggests consuming limited amounts of dairy, eggs, and animal proteins. The diet places a strong emphasis on consuming organic, non-GMO foods and local, seasonal produce.

The Apple Crisp Pegan Diet promotes the consumption of healthy fats from sources like olive oil, coconut oil, and avocado in addition to its emphasis on plant-based meals. It also suggests consuming whole grains, fruits, and vegetables as well as other wholesome forms of carbs.

Eating foods with less processing and devoid of additives and preservatives is highly prioritized on the Apple Crisp Pegan Diet. Additionally, it advises staying away from foods that have been through a lot of processing and sugar.

The Apple Crisp Pegan Diet's great flexibility allows it to be customized to suit each person's preferences and requirements, which is one of its key benefits. Additionally, it can be modified to accommodate various lifestyles, including those of athletes, vegans, and those with specific nutritional needs.

An excellent way to develop and keep up a healthy lifestyle is the Apple Crisp Pegan diet. It promotes the consumption of nutrient-dense, whole foods and is sustainable and balanced. The Paleo and vegan diets are the foundation of the diet, and it combines elements of both to produce a balanced and nutrient-rich way of living. If you want to develop and maintain a healthy lifestyle, the Apple Crisp Pegan Diet is a great option.

PRINCIPLE 2: PALEO BROWNIES

WHAT IS PALEO DIET?

A dietary regimen focused on the kinds of food that are thought to have been consumed by early humans during the Paleolithic epoch is known as the Paleo Diet, often referred to as the Caveman Diet. This diet excludes all foods that became accessible after the advent of agriculture and only includes items that were available during the Paleolithic epoch. Grain, legumes, dairy products, and processed foods are all included in this. Lean proteins, produce, nuts, and seeds, together with fruits and vegetables, make up the bulk of the diet.

The Paleo diet's major objective is to encourage individuals to eat more naturally occurring, unprocessed foods while minimizing their consumption of processed foods, which are believed to be the root cause of many current health problems. This eating plan is said to improve digestion, lessen inflammation, and advance general health and wellness.

WHAT IS PALEO BROWNIE?

Paleo Brownies are a particular kind of dessert that are produced with Paleo-friendly ingredients. There are no grains, dairy products, or refined sugars used in the preparation of Paleo brownies. As a base, they frequently start with nut flours like almond, coconut, or hazelnut flour before being sweetened with honey or maple syrup. They can also be prepared without using additional fats like butter or oil.

Paleo brownies are a wonderful way to enjoy a sweet treat without compromising your dedication to the Paleo Diet. They serve as a healthier substitute for conventional brownies, which are typically produced with grains, dairy products, and refined sugars.

PALEO BROWNIES' PERKS

The Paleo Diet has many advantages, and Paleo Brownies are no exception. These are a few of the main advantages:

1. Little Additional Sugar: Conventional brownies include refined sugar, which can induce blood sugar rises and has no nutritious value. Paleo brownies don't contain any additional sugar and are produced with natural sweeteners like honey or maple syrup.

2. High in Fiber: Nut flours, which are a good source of dietary fiber, are a common ingredient in Paleo brownie recipes. Fiber can help to regulate your digestive system and keeps you full for longer.

3. High in Healthy Fats: Nut butters, which are a wonderful source of healthy fats, are a common ingredient in Paleo brownie recipes. A good diet must include healthy fats because they provide you energy and assist to control your hormones.

4. Gluten-Free: Paleo brownies are a terrific choice for anyone who are sensitive to or intolerant of gluten because they don't contain any grains that carry gluten.

5. Low Calorie: Paleo Brownies often have fewer calories than regular brownies. They are therefore a fantastic choice for anybody trying to limit their calorie consumption.

PALEO BROWNIE MAKING INSTRUCTIONS

Paleo brownies are simple to make and only require a few straightforward steps. The following is a basic Paleo brownie recipe:

Ingredients:

almond flour, 1 cup

a half-cup of cocoa powder

A half-teaspoon of baking powder

14 teaspoons of salt

Honey, 1/4 cup

a quarter cup of melted coconut oil

2 eggs

Vanilla extract, 1 teaspoon

Instructions:

1. Set oven temperature to 350°F (175°C).

2. Use coconut oil to grease an 8x8-inch baking tray.

3. Combine the almond flour, salt, baking soda, and cocoa powder in a big bowl.

4. Combine honey, melted coconut oil, eggs, and vanilla extract in another bowl.

5. Add the wet ingredients to the dry ones and stir to incorporate.

6. Spoon the batter evenly into the baking pan.

7. Bake for 25 to 30 minutes, or until a toothpick inserted comes out clean.

8. Let the food cool completely before cutting into squares.

CONCLUSION

Paleo brownies are a wonderful way to enjoy a sweet treat without compromising your dedication to the Paleo Diet. These brownies are a wonderful source of nutritional fiber, healthy fats, and antioxidants and are created without the use of grains, dairy products, or processed sweets. They are a healthy choice for people wanting to limit their calorie or gluten intake because they are likewise low in calories and gluten-free. Paleo brownies are simple to make and only require a few straightforward steps. Therefore, give cooking some Paleo Brownies a try today if you're seeking for a tasty and nutritious dessert.

PRINCIPLE #3

INTRODUCTION
COCONUT MACAROONS FOR A PEGAN DIET

Since ancient times, coconut macaroons have been a popular sweet treat that has delighted palates everywhere with its sweet coconut flavor and chewy texture. A common food on many diets, especially the Paleo and vegan diets, is the coconut macaroon. We will look at how the coconut macaroon fits into the Pegan diet, which combines the Paleo and vegan diets, in this book. We'll go over the coconut macaroon's nutritional profile, how it may be included into a Pegan diet, and several delectable coconut macaroon dishes.

A COCONUT MACAROON IS WHAT?

Coconut, sugar, and egg whites are used to make the sweet treat known as a coconut macaroon. After combining the ingredients, they are baked in the oven. A chewy, sweet delight that is adored worldwide is the end product. Numerous nations, notably the French, Italians, and Jews, have relished coconut macaroons for generations.

VALUE OF NUTRITION IN COCONUT MACAROONS

Coconut macaroons contain a number of important vitamins and minerals. They are a good source of dietary fiber, which is crucial for regularity and digestive health. Iron, magnesium, phosphorus, potassium, zinc, and manganese are additional nutrients found in coconut macaroons. Additionally, they are a good source of monounsaturated and polyunsaturated fatty acids, which are good for the heart.

With roughly 3 grams per serving, coconut macaroons are a fantastic source of protein as well. They are therefore a fantastic snack for vegans and people following a Pegan diet. With only 150 calories per serving, coconut macaroons are extremely calorie-efficient.

HOW TO INCLUDE COCONUT MACARONS IN A VEGETARIAN DIET.

A Pegan diet, which combines the Paleo and vegan diets, might include coconut macaroons as a treat. A key component of the Paleo diet is consuming complete, unprocessed foods that are rich in protein, fiber, and healthy fats. Eating plant-based foods, such as fruits, vegetables, grains, legumes, nuts, and seeds, is the main component of the vegan diet.

With a focus on eating complete, unprocessed foods that are high in fiber and plant-based proteins, the Pegan diet blends these two eating patterns. Due to their low calorie content, good fat content, and protein content, coconut macaroons can be included in a Pegan diet. They can also be savored guilt-free as a sweet treat!

YUMMY RECIPES FOR COCONUT MACAROONS

Here are some mouthwatering coconut macaroon recipes that are suitable for a Pegan diet.

Traditional Coconut Macarons

Ingredients:

3 cups of unsweetened coconut sugar, 2/3 cup of coconut sugar, and 3 egg whites.

1/2 teaspoon vanilla essence and 1/4 teaspoon salt

Instructions:

1. Set the oven to 350 degrees.

2. Combine the coconut, coconut sugar, salt, and vanilla essence in a sizable bowl.

3. Whip the egg whites in a another basin until frothy.

4. Gently combine the coconut mixture with the egg whites.

5. Use parchment paper to cover a baking sheet.

6. Using a scoop, drop the mixture onto the baking sheet, leaving space between scoops.

7. Bake for 12 to 15 minutes, or until the top is golden.

Let the food cool before serving. Enjoy!

Macaroons with chocolate and coconut

Ingredients:

3 cups of unsweetened coconut sugar and 2/3 cup of coconut milk

three egg whites

1 teaspoon vanilla extract, 1/4 teaspoon salt, and 1/3 cup dark chocolate chips.

INSTRUCTIONS:

1. Set the oven to 350 degrees.

2. Combine the coconut, coconut sugar, salt, and vanilla essence in a sizable bowl.

3. Whip the egg whites in a another basin until frothy.

4. Gently combine the coconut mixture with the egg whites.

5. Include the dark chocolate chunks and mix well.

6. Use parchment paper to cover a baking sheet.

7. Place a gap between each scoop of the mixture as you place it on the baking sheet.

8. Bake for 12 to 15 minutes, or until the top is golden.

9. Wait until cool before serving. Enjoy!

CONCLUSION

A sweet treat you can enjoy as part of a Pegan diet are coconut macaroons. In addition to offering some protein and good fats, they are low in calories and a good source of dietary fiber. With any luck, these recipes have given you the motivation to make coconut macaroons at home and incorporate them into your Pegan diet. Good appetite!

BENEFITS TO HEALTH OF THIS DIET

The Pegan Diet places a strong emphasis on consuming complete, unprocessed foods that are nutrient-dense. This kind of diet is loaded with healthy fats, fiber, protein, and vitamins and minerals. This type of eating can aid in promoting weight loss, reducing inflammation, and enhancing general health. A healthy gut flora can be supported by plant-based proteins, which are encouraged by the Pegan Diet. A diet high in fiber and plant-based proteins can also decrease blood pressure and cholesterol.

50 FACTS ABOUT THE PEGAN DIET

1. The Pegan diet combines the vegan and paleo diets.

2. It promotes a diet high in fruits, vegetables, nuts, and seeds that is based on plants.

3. It also permits a limited quantity of animal protein from sources including fish, poultry, and eggs.

4. It's intended to encourage weight loss and enhance general wellness.

5. The Pegan diet forbids eating refined and processed foods.

6. It emphasizes wholesome, unprocessed foods high in vitamins, minerals, and good fats.

7. These consist of whole grains, nuts, seeds, legumes, fruits, vegetables, and healthy oils.

8. It also permits the moderate consumption of lean proteins including fish, chicken, and eggs.

9. It is best to avoid red meat, dairy products, and processed meats.

10. Refined carbohydrates and sugary drinks like soda and energy drinks are also forbidden.

11. The Pegan diet has a low caloric intake by nature.

12. It lowers the risk of chronic diseases and inflammation.

13. A lot of fruits, vegetables, and nuts should be consumed.

14. Moderate amounts of animal protein are permitted.

15. It discourages the consumption of refined and processed foods as well as sugary drinks.

16. It can aid in losing weight and enhancing general health.

17. It is a wholesome and well-balanced diet.

18. It emphasizes whole, nutrient-dense foods.

19. It contains a lot of healthy fats, vitamins, and minerals.

It promotes minimizing intake of processed meals and animal proteins.

It places a focus on consuming whole, unprocessed foods.

22. It may aid in lowering body inflammation.

23. It encourages better eating practices.

24. It has few calories by nature.

25. It can lower the risk of developing chronic illnesses like diabetes and heart disease.

26. It supports maintaining the body's equilibrium.

It supports consuming a variety of whole foods.

It aids in maintaining a healthy weight (number 28).

29. It might increase vigor.

30. It is stocked with wholesome and delectable dishes.

It is predicated on the idea that the majority of processed and refined meals ought to be avoided.

32. It may be useful in lowering cravings for unhealthy meals.

33. It promotes a healthy eating philosophy.

It permits modest amounts of animal protein, including that found in fish and eggs.

Red meat, dairy products, and processed meats are discouraged.

36. It might aid in lowering the risk of obesity.

37. It places a strong emphasis on consuming foods high in fiber.

38. It may aid with digestive improvement.

It aids in lowering cholesterol levels, number 39.

It promotes intentional and mindful eating.

41. It assists in controlling blood sugar levels.

It emphasizes consuming wholesome, nutritious foods.

43. It may help to reduce the chance of developing some cancers.

44. It can aid in enhancing mental acuity and concentration.

It may aid in lowering stress levels.

46. It may aid in lowering the chance of developing heart disease.

47. It may aid in elevating mood and energy levels.

It is predicated on consuming a variety of nutrient-rich foods.

49. It promotes mindful eating and portion control.

50. It may contribute to bettering general health and happiness.

PEGAN DIET IS IT KETO?

The Pegan diet is not a ketogenic one. Both diets emphasize consuming whole, unprocessed foods that are high in nutrients, but the Pegan diet permits a small amount of animal protein and a moderate amount of carbohydrates, whereas the keto diet forgoes most carbohydrates and concentrates on high-fat foods.

CONCLUSION

A combination of the Paleo and vegan diets, the Pegan diet places a strong emphasis on a plant-based diet that includes lots of fruits, vegetables, nuts, and seeds as well as a moderate amount of animal protein. This diet is intended to encourage weight loss, enhance general health, and lessen inflammatory responses within the body. The Pegan diet avoids processed foods, red meat, dairy products, and sugar in favor of whole, unprocessed foods that are high in vitamins, minerals, and healthy fats. This type of eating plan aids in weight loss, health improvement, and the reduction of inflammation.

The Pegan diet is an eating plan that emphasizes whole, nutrient-dense foods that are already low in calories. It forbids red meat, dairy, and processed foods while permitting moderate amounts of lean proteins from sources like poultry, eggs, and fish. Refined cereals and sweetened beverages are also forbidden. People can enhance their health, lessen inflammation, and reduce weight by adopting the Pegan diet.